CHAPTER 1

WHAT IS THE PSMF DIET?

Definition of PSMF (Protein-Sparing Modified Fast) Diet

The Protein-Sparing Modified Fast (PSMF) diet is a specialized and structured diet plan that focuses on maximizing weight loss while minimizing muscle loss. It is a short-term, medically supervised diet typically recommended for individuals who are significantly overweight or obese and need to lose weight quickly for health reasons.

The PSMF diet is characterized by its high protein intake and severely restricted calorie consumption. The primary objective is to provide the body with sufficient protein while minimizing overall caloric intake. By doing so, the diet aims to preserve lean body mass (muscle) while promoting fat loss.

The term "protein-sparing" in PSMF refers to the idea that adequate protein intake protects the body from breaking down muscle tissue for energy. Instead, the body primarily relies on stored fat for fuel, leading to rapid weight loss.

Purpose and Benefits of the PSMF Diet

The PSMF diet serves several purposes and offers various benefits for individuals looking to lose weight efficiently and effectively. Here are some of the key reasons why people may choose to follow a PSMF diet:

1. Rapid Weight Loss: The PSMF diet is designed to induce rapid weight loss, typically between 4 to 7 pounds per week. This quick initial progress can provide a motivational boost, making it easier for individuals to stick to the diet plan.

2. Muscle Preservation: Unlike traditional low-calorie diets, the PSMF diet aims to preserve lean body mass. The high protein content supports muscle maintenance and prevents muscle breakdown, which can be common during periods of calorie restriction.

3. Metabolic Reset: The PSMF diet helps reset the body's metabolism by encouraging it to primarily burn stored fat for energy. This can be beneficial for individuals with slow metabolisms or those who have reached a weight loss plateau.

4. Improved Insulin Sensitivity: The PSMF diet may enhance insulin sensitivity, which is beneficial for individuals with insulin resistance or type 2 diabetes. By reducing overall caloric intake and promoting weight loss, the diet can help regulate blood sugar levels.

5. Structured Approach: The PSMF diet provides a structured and controlled approach to weight loss. It involves carefully calculated macronutrient ratios and portion sizes, making it easier for individuals to adhere to the diet plan.

6. Motivation and Discipline: Following a strict and regimented diet like PSMF requires discipline and commitment. For some individuals, this level of structure can be motivating and empowering, leading to a sense of control over their eating habits.

Overview of How the PSMF Diet Works

The PSMF diet works by creating a significant caloric deficit while maintaining adequate protein intake. Here is a step-by-step overview of how the PSMF diet typically operates:

1. **Calculating Protein Intake:** The first step in the PSMF diet is determining the appropriate protein intake for an individual. This is usually based on lean body mass, and the recommended daily protein intake typically ranges between 0.6 to 1 gram of protein per pound of lean body mass.

2. **Severe Caloric Restriction:** The total caloric intake on the PSMF diet is extremely low, typically ranging between 500 to 800 calories per day. These calories primarily come from lean protein sources.

3. **Minimal Carbohydrate and Fat Intake:** Carbohydrate and fat consumption is severely limited on the PSMF diet. The diet focuses on lean protein sources such as skinless chicken breast, fish, lean cuts of meat, and low-fat dairy products.

4. **Supplementation:** Due to the significant calorie restriction, individuals following the PSMF diet may require vitamin and mineral supplementation to ensure they receive essential nutrients. This is important to prevent deficiencies and support overall health during the period of caloric restriction.

5. **Strict Meal Planning:** Following the PSMF diet requires careful meal planning to ensure that the limited calories are distributed appropriately

throughout the day. Meals are often small and frequent, with an emphasis on lean protein sources and low-calorie vegetables.

6. **Medical Supervision:** The PSMF diet is typically recommended under medical supervision to ensure safety and monitor progress. Regular check-ups, blood tests, and consultations with healthcare professionals are important to assess the individual's response to the diet and make any necessary adjustments.

7. **Limited Duration:** The PSMF diet is not meant to be followed long-term. It is considered a short-term intervention, usually lasting between 2 to 12 weeks, depending on individual goals and medical considerations. After completing the PSMF diet, individuals are advised to transition to a more sustainable and balanced eating plan.

8. **Exercise Recommendations:** While exercise is not a mandatory component of the PSMF diet, light to moderate physical activity is often encouraged. This helps maintain muscle mass, supports overall health, and can aid in weight loss. However, intense or strenuous exercise may not be suitable during the period of severe caloric restriction.

It's important to note that the PSMF diet is not suitable for everyone. It is typically recommended for individuals who are significantly overweight or obese and need to lose weight rapidly for medical reasons. It should only be undertaken under the guidance of healthcare professionals experienced in administering this type of diet.

UNDERSTANDING MACRONUTRIENTS

Explanation of Macronutrients (Protein, Carbohydrates, and Fat)

Macronutrients are the essential nutrients required by the body in large quantities to support various bodily functions, energy production, and overall well-being. The three primary macronutrients are protein, carbohydrates, and fat. Each macronutrient plays a unique role in our diet and has distinct effects on our bodies.

Protein is often considered the building block of life. It is composed of amino acids and is crucial for the growth, repair, and maintenance of tissues, including muscles, organs, and skin. Protein also plays a vital role in the production of enzymes, hormones, and antibodies. Dietary sources of protein include lean meats, poultry, fish, dairy products, legumes, nuts, and seeds.

Carbohydrates are the body's primary source of energy. They are broken down into glucose, which is used by cells for fuel. Carbohydrates can be further classified into two main types: simple carbohydrates and complex carbohydrates. Simple carbohydrates, found in fruits, vegetables, and refined sugars, provide quick bursts of energy. Complex carbohydrates, found in whole grains, legumes, and starchy vegetables, release energy more gradually and help maintain steady blood sugar levels.

Fat is often misunderstood as being unhealthy, but it is an essential nutrient for our bodies. Fat provides energy, helps in the absorption of fat-soluble vitamins (such as vitamins A, D, E, and K), and aids in the production of hormones. There are different types of dietary fats, including saturated fats, unsaturated fats (monounsaturated and polyunsaturated fats), and trans fats. Saturated fats, found in animal products and some plant oils, should be consumed in moderation. Unsaturated fats, found in nuts, seeds, avocados, and fatty fish, are considered healthier options. Trans fats, found in processed and fried foods, should be avoided as much as possible.

A well-balanced diet includes an appropriate combination of macronutrients. The ideal macronutrient distribution varies depending on individual factors such as age, sex, activity level, and overall health goals. It is generally recommended that protein intake should make up about 10-35% of total daily calories, carbohydrates should contribute 45-65%, and fat should account for 20-35%. However, specific dietary needs may differ, and it's best to consult with a healthcare professional or registered dietitian for personalized recommendations.

Importance of Protein in the PSMF Diet

The Protein-Sparing Modified Fast (PSMF) diet is a specialized approach to weight loss that prioritizes protein intake while severely limiting carbohydrates and fat consumption. This diet is often utilized under medical supervision for individuals who are obese or need to lose weight rapidly, such as before surgery. Protein plays a crucial role in the PSMF diet for several reasons.

1. **Preservation of Lean Muscle Mass:** During periods of significant calorie restriction, the body may turn to its own muscle tissue as a source of energy. Adequate protein intake helps minimize muscle breakdown and preserves lean muscle mass, which is important for maintaining metabolic rate and overall strength.

2. **Increased Satiety and Reduced Hunger:** Protein is known to promote feelings of fullness and satiety. By including sufficient protein in the PSMF diet, individuals are more likely to feel satisfied and less inclined to overeat or snack between meals. This can be particularly helpful during a calorie-restricted diet.

3. **Thermic Effect of Food (TEF):** Protein has a higher thermic effect compared to carbohydrates and fats. The thermic effect refers to the increase in energy expenditure during the digestion, absorption, and processing of nutrients. By consuming more protein in the PSMF diet, individuals can potentially increase their overall energy expenditure and enhance fat burning.

4. **Maintenance of Metabolic Rate:** When the body is subjected to a significant calorie deficit, there is a risk of metabolic rate slowing down. This can hinder weight loss progress. Protein has a higher thermic effect and helps maintain metabolic rate by supporting muscle mass. By prioritizing protein intake, the PSMF diet aims to mitigate the decrease in metabolic rate that can occur during weight loss.

5. **Nutrient Density:** Protein-rich foods are often

nutrient-dense, meaning they provide a wide range of essential vitamins, minerals, and amino acids. While the PSMF diet restricts overall calorie intake, ensuring an adequate intake of essential nutrients is crucial. Protein sources such as lean meats, fish, poultry, eggs, and low-fat dairy products can contribute to meeting these nutrient needs.

6. **Muscle Repair and Recovery:** In addition to preserving muscle mass, protein plays a vital role in the repair and recovery of muscles. For individuals who engage in regular physical activity or exercise while following the PSMF diet, protein becomes even more important. It helps repair damaged muscle tissue, supports optimal muscle function, and aids in post-workout recovery.

It is essential to note that the PSMF diet is a short-term and highly restrictive approach to weight loss. It should only be undertaken under medical supervision and for a specific duration. Prolonged adherence to a PSMF diet may lead to nutrient deficiencies and other health risks. Once the desired weight loss goal is achieved, transitioning to a more balanced and sustainable eating plan is crucial for long-term health and weight management.

Role of Carbohydrates and Fat in the PSMF Diet

While the PSMF diet emphasizes high protein intake, it significantly restricts carbohydrates and fat consumption. Carbohydrates and fat still have important roles to play in the overall function of the body, and understanding their role in the PSMF diet is essential.

1. **Carbohydrates:** Carbohydrates are the body's

primary source of energy, particularly for intense physical activities and brain function. In the PSMF diet, carbohydrates are severely limited to induce a state of ketosis. Ketosis is a metabolic state where the body primarily relies on fat for fuel because carbohydrate stores are depleted. By restricting carbohydrates, the PSMF diet aims to promote the breakdown of stored body fat for energy, leading to rapid weight loss.

2. **Fat:** While fat is restricted in the PSMF diet, it still serves important functions in the body. Dietary fat provides essential fatty acids, which are necessary for various bodily processes, including hormone production, brain function, and cellular health. Fat also aids in the absorption of fat-soluble vitamins and helps maintain healthy skin and hair. In the context of the PSMF diet, the restriction of dietary fat encourages the body to utilize stored fat for energy, facilitating weight loss.

It's important to note that the severe restriction of carbohydrates and fat in the PSMF diet is not suitable for everyone, especially for those with certain medical conditions. Carbohydrates and fats are essential macronutrients that provide various health benefits, and a balanced intake is necessary for overall well-being. Once the PSMF diet phase is complete, gradually reintroducing carbohydrates and fats into the diet, while maintaining a calorie-controlled approach, can help achieve a more sustainable and balanced eating pattern.

PRINCIPLES OF THE PSMF DIET

Caloric Restriction and Aggressive Fat Loss

Caloric restriction is a dietary approach that involves reducing the number of calories consumed to create a calorie deficit, ultimately leading to weight loss. When taken to an extreme level, it can be referred to as aggressive fat loss. This approach aims to expedite fat loss by significantly reducing calorie intake. While it may produce quick results, it's important to approach aggressive fat loss with caution and prioritize long-term sustainability and overall health.

1. The concept of caloric restriction: Caloric restriction is based on the principle that when you consume fewer calories than your body needs, it will tap into its energy reserves, which include fat stores. By consistently maintaining a calorie deficit, you can promote fat loss and achieve your desired body composition goals. However, it's crucial to strike a balance between caloric restriction and providing your body with essential nutrients.

2. Determining the appropriate caloric deficit: Aggressive fat loss involves creating a more significant calorie deficit than what is typically recommended for gradual weight loss. To determine the appropriate deficit, it's essential to consider factors such as your current body weight, activity level, and metabolism. It's generally recommended to aim for a deficit of 20-30% below your maintenance calorie level, but it's advisable to consult with a healthcare professional or registered dietitian to develop a personalized plan.

3. Potential benefits and considerations: Aggressive fat loss can lead to rapid weight loss, which can be motivating for some individuals. However, it's important to approach this approach with caution and consider the potential drawbacks. Severely restricting calories for an extended period can impact energy levels, metabolism, and overall well-being. It's essential to monitor your body's response and make adjustments accordingly to ensure you're still meeting your nutritional needs.

4. Balancing macronutrients during aggressive fat loss: While creating a calorie deficit is the primary focus during aggressive fat loss, it's equally important to pay attention to macronutrient distribution. Ensuring an adequate intake of protein, carbohydrates, and fats can support muscle preservation, energy levels, and overall health. Prioritize nutrient-dense foods to meet your body's requirements and consider consulting a professional to determine the optimal macronutrient ratios for your specific goals.

5. Monitoring progress and adjusting accordingly: Regular monitoring of progress is crucial during aggressive fat loss. This includes tracking body weight, body measurements, and overall well-being. If you notice negative effects such as extreme fatigue, dizziness, or significant muscle loss, it may be necessary to reassess your approach. Adjusting the caloric deficit or macronutrient ratios may be required to strike a better balance between aggressive fat loss and overall health.

In summary, aggressive fat loss through caloric restriction can be an effective approach to expedite weight loss. However, it's crucial to prioritize overall health and sustainability. Consultation with healthcare professionals or registered dietitians is highly recommended to develop a personalized plan that meets your nutritional needs while still allowing for aggressive fat loss.

Maintaining High Protein Intake

Protein is an essential macronutrient that plays a crucial role in numerous bodily functions, including muscle repair and growth, hormone production, and immune function. Maintaining a high protein intake is important, especially during weight loss or muscle-building phases. Let's delve deeper into the significance of high protein intake and how it can benefit your overall health and fitness goals.

1. The role of protein in the body: Protein serves as the building block for various tissues, enzymes, and hormones in the body. It plays a vital role in muscle repair and growth, making it particularly important for individuals engaged in resistance training or physical activity. Additionally, protein can promote feelings of satiety, which can aid in weight management byreducing cravings and overeating.

2. Protein and weight management: High protein intake can support weight management efforts in several ways. Firstly, protein has a higher thermic effect of food compared to carbohydrates and fats, meaning that the body expends more energy to digest and process it. This can slightly increase calorie expenditure and contribute to overall energy balance. Additionally, protein helps to preserve lean muscle mass during weight loss, which is essential for maintaining a healthy metabolism. By preserving muscle mass, you can enhance your body's ability to burn calories and promote fat loss.

3. Muscle recovery and growth: For individuals engaged in regular physical activity or resistance training, protein is essential for muscle recovery and growth. During exercise, muscle fibers experience micro-tears, and adequate protein intake supports the repair and rebuilding of these tissues. Consuming protein-rich foods or supplements post-workout can optimize the recovery process and enhance muscle protein synthesis. This can lead to improved strength, performance, and body composition.

4. Satiation and appetite control: Including protein-rich foods in your meals and snacks can contribute to feelings of satiety and help control appetite. Protein takes longer to digest compared to carbohydrates, which means it can help you feel fuller for a longer period. By incorporating protein into your meals, you may be less likely to experience cravings and overeat, ultimately supporting your weight management goals.

5. Sources of high-quality protein: It's important to choose high-quality protein sources that provide essential amino acids and other nutrients. Animal-based proteins such as lean meats, poultry, fish, eggs, and dairy products are considered complete proteins as they contain all the essential amino acids. For individuals following a vegetarian or vegan diet, plant-based protein sources like legumes, tofu, tempeh, quinoa, and chia seeds can be combined to ensure an adequate amino acid profile.

6. Determining protein requirements: The recommended protein intake varies depending on factors such as age, sex, activity level, and goals. While there isn't a one-size-fits-all approach, a general guideline is to consume around 0.8-1 gram of protein per kilogram of body weight. However, individuals engaged in intense physical activity or strength training may require higher protein intake, ranging from 1.2-2.0 grams per kilogram of body weight. It's advisable to consult with a registered dietitian or healthcare professional to determine the optimal protein intake for your specific needs.

In conclusion, maintaining a high protein intake is crucial for supporting muscle repair and growth, promoting satiety, and optimizing weight management efforts. Including a variety of protein sources in your diet and tailoring your intake to your individual needs can help you achieve your health and fitness goals effectively.

Monitoring and Adjusting Macronutrient Ratios

Macronutrients, including carbohydrates, proteins, and fats, are the main sources of energy in our diet. The ratios in which we consume these macronutrients can have a significant impact on our overall health, body composition, and performance. Monitoring and adjusting macronutrient ratios can help optimize nutrition and support various goals, such as weight loss, muscle gain, or athletic performance.

1. **Understanding macronutrients:** Carbohydrates, proteins, and fats are macronutrients that provide energy and play distinct roles in the body. Carbohydrates are the primary fuel source for energy production, proteins are essential for muscle repair and growth, and fats contribute to hormone production and provide insulation for organs. Each macronutrient has a specific caloric value: carbohydrates and proteins provide 4 calories per gram, while fats provide 9 calories per gram.

2. Determining macronutrient ratios: The ideal macronutrient ratio varies depending on individual factors such as activity level, goals, and personal preferences. There is no one-size-fits-all approach, and it's important to find a balance that works best for you. Here are a few common macronutrient ratios for different goals:

- Balanced Diet: A balanced macronutrient ratio is typically composed of approximately 40-60% carbohydrates, 20-30% fats, and 20-30% proteins. This ratio is often recommended for overall health, providing a good mix of energy, essential nutrients, and promoting satiety.

- Low-Carb Diet: Low-carb diets typically involve reducing carbohydrate intake and increasing protein and fat consumption. This approach aims to shift the body into a state of ketosis, where it primarily relies on fat for fuel. Macronutrient ratios for a low-carb diet can range from 10-30% carbohydrates, 40-50% fats, and 20-30% proteins.

- High-Protein Diet: For individuals focused on muscle gain or fat loss, a higher protein intake may be beneficial. In this case, the macronutrient ratio might consist of 40-50% carbohydrates, 25-35% fats, and 25-35% proteins. This higher protein intake supports muscle repair and growth while providing adequate energy from carbohydrates and fats.

3. Monitoring macronutrient intake: To effectively monitor macronutrient ratios, it's important to track your food intake and calculate the percentage of calories coming from each macronutrient. This can be done using various apps or online tools that allow you to log your meals and provide detailed nutritional information. Regular monitoring helps ensure that you're staying within your desired macronutrient ranges and can provide insights into how different ratios impact your progress.

4. Adjusting macronutrient ratios: Macronutrient ratios are not set in stone and can be adjusted based on individual needs and goals. It's essential to listen to your body and make adjustments as necessary. For example, if you find that you're lacking energy during workouts, you may need to increase your carbohydrate intake. Similarly, if you're not seeing desired muscle gains, adjusting protein intake upwards may be beneficial.

5. Individual variations and experimentation: It's worth noting that individual variations exist when it comes to macronutrient ratios. Some individuals may thrive on a higher-carbohydrate diet, while others may feel better on a lower-carbohydrate approach. It's important to experiment and find the ratio that works best for your body and supports your goals. Consulting with a registered dietitian or nutritionist can provide valuable guidance and personalized recommendations.

In conclusion, monitoring and adjusting macronutrient ratios can help optimize your nutrition and support specific goals. By finding the right balance of carbohydrates, proteins, and fats, you can enhance energy levels, support muscle growth or weight loss, and improve overall performance and well-being. Regular monitoring and adjustments based on individual responses are key to finding the optimal macronutrient ratio for your body.

Importance of Regular Exercise

Regular exercise is a fundamental component of a healthy lifestyle, offering numerous physical and mental health benefits. Engaging in consistent physical activity can improve cardiovascular health, enhance strength and endurance, boost mood, and help maintain a healthy body weight. Let's explore the importance of regular exercise in more detail.

1. Cardiovascular health: Regular exercise, particularly aerobic activities like jogging, cycling, or swimming, can improve cardiovascular health. It strengthens the heart muscle, enhances circulation, and lowers blood pressure. Engaging in aerobic exercises increases heart rate, improving oxygen delivery to the muscles and organs, and reducing the risk of cardiovascular diseases such as heart attacks, stroke, and high cholesterol.

2. Weight management and metabolism: Exercise plays a vital role in weight management by helping to maintain a healthy body weight and supporting metabolism. Physical activity helps burn calories, contributing to a calorie deficit when combined with a balanced diet. It also promotes the development of lean muscle mass, which increases the body's metabolic rate. Regular exercise can help prevent weight gain, facilitate weight loss, and improve body composition by reducing body fat and increasing muscle tone.

3. Bone health: Weight-bearing exercises such as walking, running, dancing, or resistance training can improve bone density and reduce the risk of osteoporosis. These activities stimulate the bones, leading to increased calcium deposition and strengthening of the skeletal system. Regular exercise, especially during childhood and adolescence, plays a crucial role in optimizing peak bone mass, which is essential for long-term bone health.

4. Mental well-being: Physical activity has a profound impact on mental health and well-being. Exercise releases endorphins, often referred to as "feel-good" hormones, which can improve mood and reduce feelings of stress, anxiety, and depression. Regular exercise is also associated with better sleep quality, increased cognitive function, and improved self-esteem. Engaging in physical activity provides a natural boost to mental and emotional well-being.

5. Disease prevention: Regular exercise has been linked to a reduced risk of chronic diseases such as type 2 diabetes, certain types of cancer, and cardiovascular diseases. Physical activity helps regulate blood sugar levels, improve insulin sensitivity, and maintain a healthy body weight, all of which contribute to lowering the risk of developing these conditions. Additionally, exercise promotes a healthy immune system, reducing the likelihood of infections and boosting overall immune function.

6. Longevity and quality of life: Leading an active lifestyle and engaging in regular exercise is associated with increased longevity and improved quality of life. Exercise helps maintain physical independence and functional abilities as we age. It enhances mobility, balance, and flexibility, reducing the risk of falls and injuries. Regular exercise also promotes better cognitive function, memory, and overall brain health, which can contribute to a higher quality of life as we get older.

7. Finding the right exercise routine: It's important to find an exercise routine that suits your preferences, interests, and individual capabilities. This can help ensure consistency and enjoyment, increasing the likelihood of maintaining a long-term exercise habit. It's recommended to include a combination of cardiovascular exercises, strength training, and flexibility exercises to achieve overall fitness and maximize the benefits.

In conclusion, regular exercise is vital for maintaining a healthy lifestyle and promoting overall well-being. Engaging in physical activity offers a wide range of benefits, including improved cardiovascular health, weight management, enhanced bone density, mental well-being, disease prevention, and increased longevity. Finding enjoyable activities and incorporating regular exercise into your daily routine can have a profound positive impact on both your physical and mental health.

SAFETY CONSIDERATIONS AND PRECAUTIONS

Potential risks and side effects of the PSMF Diet

The Protein-Sparing Modified Fast (PSMF) diet is a highly restrictive and low-calorie diet that primarily focuses on protein intake while severely limiting carbohydrate and fat consumption. While the PSMF diet may lead to rapid weight loss, it's important to be aware of potential risks and side effects associated with this approach.

1. **Nutrient deficiencies:** The PSMF diet restricts the intake of various food groups, which may result in inadequate nutrient intake. Since the diet is low in carbohydrates and fats, it may be challenging to obtain essential vitamins, minerals, and dietary fiber. Long-term adherence to this diet without proper supplementation may lead to deficiencies in nutrients such as vitamins A, D, E, and K, as well as calcium, magnesium, and potassium.

2. **Muscle loss:** Although the PSMF diet is designed to spare muscle tissue by providing a high protein intake, there is still a risk of muscle loss due to the severe calorie restriction. Consuming too few

calories for an extended period can result in the body breaking down muscle tissue for energy. To minimize muscle loss, it's crucial to ensure an adequate protein intake and engage in resistance training exercises.

3. **Metabolic adaptations:** Prolonged adherence to the PSMF diet can lead to metabolic adaptations. The body may adjust to the reduced calorie intake by slowing down metabolism to conserve energy. This can make weight loss more challenging and lead to weight regain once normal eating habits are resumed.

4. **Gallstone formation:** Rapid weight loss, which can occur on the PSMF diet, has been associated with an increased risk of gallstone formation. Gallstones are hardened deposits that can block the bile ducts, causing severe pain and potentially requiring medical intervention. It's important to consult with a healthcare professional before starting this diet, especially if you have a history of gallbladder or liver problems.

5. **Digestive issues:** The PSMF diet may cause digestive discomfort, including constipation, as it lacks dietary fiber from carbohydrates. Insufficient fiber intake can lead to irregular bowel movements and potentially contribute to gastrointestinal issues. It's important to ensure adequate hydration and consider incorporating low-carbohydrate sources of fiber, such as non-starchy vegetables, to mitigate these effects.

6. **Psychological impact:** The highly restrictive nature of the PSMF diet can have psychological

implications, particularly for individuals prone to disordered eating patterns or those with a history of eating disorders. The strict limitations and monotony of the diet may increase the risk of developing an unhealthy relationship with food or trigger feelings of guilt or anxiety around eating.

To minimize the risks and side effects associated with the PSMF diet, it's crucial to approach it with caution and under the guidance of a healthcare professional. Individual factors such as overall health, medical history, and current medications should be taken into consideration. Additionally, it's important to follow the diet for a limited duration and cycle it with periods of balanced nutrition to mitigate potential long-term health risks. Regular monitoring of health markers and close supervision by a healthcare professional is essential to ensure the diet is being implemented safely and effectively.

Who should avoid or approach the PSMF Diet with caution?

While the PSMF diet may be effective for certain individuals, it is not suitable or recommended for everyone. Specific groups of individuals should avoid or approach the PSMF diet with caution due to potential health risks and complications. It's important to consider the following factors:

1. **Pregnant or breastfeeding women:** During pregnancy and lactation, adequate nutrition is essential for the health of both the mother and the child. The PSMF diet's severe calorie restriction and potential nutrient deficiencies make it unsuitable for these stages of life

2. **Individuals with underlying health conditions:** People with pre-existing health conditions such as diabetes, kidney disease, liver disease, cardiovascular disease, or any metabolic disorders should exercise caution when considering the PSMF diet. The severe calorie restriction and specific nutrient composition of the diet may not provide the necessary nutrients to support their overall health and may exacerbate their condition.

3. **Elderly individuals:** Older adults often have different nutritional needs due to changes in metabolism and potential age-related health issues. The PSMF diet's restrictive nature may increase the risk of nutrient deficiencies and muscle loss in this population. It is crucial for elderly individuals to prioritize a well-rounded, balanced diet that meets their specific nutrient requirements.

4. **Individuals with a history of eating disorders:** Those with a history of eating disorders, such as anorexia nervosa or bulimia, should avoid the PSMF diet. The highly restrictive nature of the diet can trigger unhealthy behaviors and exacerbate psychological stress surrounding food. It's essential for individuals with a history of disordered eating to focus on nourishing their bodies in a balanced and sustainable way.

5. **Athletes or individuals with high physical activity levels:** Individuals who engage in intense physical activity or have high energy demands may not find the PSMF diet suitable for their

needs. The low calorie and carbohydrate content of the diet may not provide enough energy to support their performance, recovery, and overall athletic goals. It is important for active individuals to prioritize a diet that provides adequate fuel for their activities.

6. **Individuals with a history of gallbladder or liver problems:** The rapid weight loss associated with the PSMF diet can increase the risk of gallstone formation, particularly in individuals who already have a history of gallbladder or liver issues. It's crucial to consult with a healthcare professional before starting this diet if you have a history of such problems.

If you fall into any of these categories, it is recommended to seek guidance from a healthcare professional or registered dietitian before considering the PSMF diet. They can help assess your individual circumstances, provide personalized recommendations, and guide you toward a more appropriate and sustainable approach to weight management and overall health.

Recommended duration and frequency of PSMF cycles

The PSMF diet is not intended to be a long-term dietary approach. It is considered an aggressive and short-term intervention for rapid weight loss or for specific medical purposes under close medical supervision. The duration and frequency of PSMF cycles can vary depending on individual goals and health considerations. Here are some general recommendations:

1. **Duration:** A typical PSMF cycle may range from 1 to 12 weeks, with 2 to 4 weeks being a commonly recommended duration. Shorter cycles are often

used for individuals with less weight to lose or those who require a shorter period of aggressive intervention. Longer cycles may be considered for individuals with significant weight to lose or for medical reasons, but should always be monitored by a healthcare professional.

2. **Maintenance periods:** It's crucial to include maintenance periods between PSMF cycles. These periods allow the body to recover, restore metabolic balance, and prevent potential long-term negative health effects. Maintenance periods typically involve gradually increasing calorie intake and transitioning to a more balanced and sustainable eating plan that meets individual nutritional needs.

3. **Individualized approach:** The duration and frequency of PSMF cycles should be tailored to each individual's specific goals, health status, and response to the diet. It is important to consult with a healthcare professional or registered dietitian to determine the appropriate duration and frequency of PSMF cycles based on your unique circumstances.

Remember that the PSMF diet should not be attempted without medical supervision or guidance. Rapid weight loss can have potential risks and side effects, and it's crucial to consult with a healthcare professional or registered dietitian who can provide personalized recommendations and monitor your progress throughout the PSMF cycles. They can help ensure that the diet is implemented safely and effectively, taking into account your individual needs and potential risks.

Consulting with a healthcare professional before starting the diet

Before embarking on any new diet or weight loss plan, including the PSMF diet, it is highly advisable to consult with a healthcare professional. Here are some reasons why seeking professional guidance is essential:

1. **Assessment of individual suitability:** A healthcare professional can assess whether the PSMF diet is appropriate for your specific needs and health status. They will consider factors such as your current weight, medical history, medications, and any underlying health conditions. They can help determine if the diet aligns with your goals and if there are any potential risks or contraindications.

2. **Monitoring overall health:** Healthcare professionals can conduct comprehensive health evaluations to ensure that you are in good overall health before starting the PSMF diet. They may perform blood tests to assess your nutrient levels, liver function, kidney function, and other relevant health markers. This can help identify any potential health risks or complications that need to be addressed before beginning the diet.

3. **Development of an individualized plan:** A healthcare professional can create a personalized PSMF plan tailored to your specific needs and goals. They will take into account factors such as your ideal caloric intake, protein requirements, nutrient needs, and any necessary modifications based on your unique circumstances. This individualized approach ensures that the diet is

optimized for your health and well-being.

4. **Monitoring and adjustments:** Regular monitoring and follow-up appointments with a healthcare professional are essential during the PSMF diet. They can track your progress, evaluate any potential side effects or complications, and make adjustments to the diet as needed. This ongoing support and supervision help ensure your safety and the effectiveness of the diet.

5. **Addressing concerns and providing guidance:** Consulting with a healthcare professional gives you the opportunity to address any concerns or questions you may have about the PSMF diet. They can provide guidance on meal planning, supplementation, managing potential side effects, and maintaining a balanced approach to nutrition and overall health.

By involving a healthcare professional in your journey with the PSMF diet, you can significantly reduce the risks associated with this highly restrictive approach. Their expertise and guidance can help ensure that you are implementing the diet safely and effectively, while also addressing any potential underlying health concerns.

In conclusion, the PSMF diet, although it can lead to rapid weight loss, carries potential risks and side effects that should be carefully considered. It is crucial to approach this diet with caution, especially if you fall into specific groups such as pregnant or breastfeeding women, individuals with underlying health conditions, the elderly, those with a history of eating disorders, athletes, or individuals with a history of gallbladder or liver problems. The duration and frequency of PSMF cycles should be personalized and monitored by a healthcare professional, and consulting with them before starting the diet is highly recommended. Their guidance can ensure your safety, minimize potential risks, and help you achieve your health goals in a sustainable manner.

STRUCTURING YOUR PSMF DIET PLAN

Determining Calorie and Protein Targets

Determining calorie and protein targets is a crucial aspect of designing a well-rounded and balanced diet plan. Calorie and protein targets are individualized and depend on factors such as age, gender, body weight, activity level, and specific goals, such as weight loss, muscle gain, or maintenance. By understanding these targets, individuals can optimize their nutrition to support overall health and achieve their desired outcomes.

Calorie Targets

Calories are a measure of energy, and determining the appropriate calorie target is essential for maintaining a healthy weight. To determine the calorie target, it is important to consider factors such as basal metabolic rate (BMR), physical activity level, and goals.

1. **Basal Metabolic Rate (BMR):** BMR refers to the number of calories your body needs to perform basic functions at rest, such as breathing and maintaining organ function. Various formulas, such as the Harris-Benedict equation, can

estimate BMR based on factors like age, gender, height, and weight.

2. **Physical Activity Level**: To determine the total calorie needs, the BMR should be multiplied by an activity factor. This factor takes into account the intensity and frequency of physical activity. Sedentary individuals have a lower activity factor, while active individuals have a higher one.

3. **Goals**: Calorie targets differ depending on whether the goal is weight loss, weight maintenance, or weight gain. To lose weight, a calorie deficit is required, which means consuming fewer calories than the body needs. Weight maintenance requires calorie balance, while weight gain necessitates a calorie surplus.

Protein Targets

Protein is an essential macronutrient that plays a vital role in numerous bodily functions, including muscle repair, growth, and hormone production. Determining the appropriate protein target ensures adequate intake to support these functions.

1. **Recommended Daily Allowance (RDA)**: The RDA for protein is approximately 0.8 grams per kilogram of body weight for adults. However, this recommendation may not be sufficient for individuals with specific goals, such as athletes or individuals undergoing resistance training. They may require a higher protein intake to support muscle protein synthesis and recovery.

2. **Specific Goals**: Depending on the individual's goals, protein intake may vary. For example,

individuals aiming for muscle gain or strength training may require higher protein targets ranging from 1.2 to 2.0 grams per kilogram of body weight. Consultation with a registered dietitian or nutritionist can help determine the appropriate protein target based on specific goals and requirements.

Dividing Meals and Snacks Throughout the Day

Dividing meals and snacks throughout the day is an effective strategy to maintain stable blood sugar levels, provide sustained energy, and prevent overeating. This approach ensures a steady supply of nutrients and helps optimize metabolism and digestion.

1. **Regular Meal Pattern**: Establishing a regular meal pattern involves consuming three main meals (breakfast, lunch, and dinner) and incorporating one or two snacks between these meals. Spacing meals and snacks evenly throughout the day helps prevent long gaps between eating, which can lead to excessive hunger and unhealthy food choices.

2. **Balanced Macronutrients**: Each meal and snack should include a balance of macronutrients, namely carbohydrates, proteins, and fats. Carbohydrates provide energy, proteins support muscle repair and growth, and fats aid in nutrient absorption and satiety. Including all three macronutrients in each eating occasion ensures a well-rounded and nutritionally complete diet.

3. **Snack Options**: Healthy snack options can include a combination of protein, complex carbohydrates, and healthy fats. Examples include

Greek yogurt with fruit, a handful of nuts and seeds, whole grain crackers with hummus, or a vegetable and protein

Balancing Macronutrients in Each Meal

Balancing macronutrients in each meal is essential for providing the body with a wide range of nutrients and maintaining overall health. Macronutrients include carbohydrates, proteins, and fats, and they all play unique roles in the body. By incorporating a balanced mix of these macronutrients into meals, individuals can optimize their nutrition and support their wellness goals.

Carbohydrates

Carbohydrates are the body's primary source of energy and should be included in each meal. They come in two forms: simple carbohydrates and complex carbohydrates.

1. **Simple Carbohydrates**: Simple carbohydrates are found in foods such as fruits, milk, and refined sugars. While they provide quick energy, they are digested rapidly and can cause blood sugar spikes. It is important to consume simple carbohydrates in moderation and choose healthier options such as whole fruits instead of sugary snacks.

2. **Complex Carbohydrates**: Complex carbohydrates are found in foods like whole grains, legumes, and vegetables. They provide sustained energy and are rich in fiber, vitamins, and minerals. Incorporating complex carbohydrates into meals helps maintain stable blood sugar levels, promotes satiety, and supports digestive health.

Proteins

Proteins are essential for the growth, repair, and

maintenance of tissues and cells in the body. They are made up of amino acids, which are the building blocks of protein. Including adequate protein in each meal is important for various bodily functions and can help individuals feel satisfied and maintain muscle mass.

1. **Lean Protein Sources**: Opt for lean protein sources such as poultry, fish, eggs, legumes, and tofu. These options provide high-quality protein with lower amounts of saturated fats. Including a variety of protein sources in meals helps ensure a diverse intake of amino acids and essential nutrients.

2. **Protein Portions**: The recommended amount of protein per meal can vary depending on factors such as age, weight, and activity level. A general guideline is to aim for 20-30 grams of protein per meal. This can be achieved by including a palm-sized portion of lean protein or incorporating protein-rich foods like Greek yogurt, cottage cheese, or nuts into meals.

Fats

Fats are an essential part of a balanced diet and provide energy, support cell growth, and help absorb fat-soluble vitamins. However, it is important to choose healthy fats and consume them in moderation.

1. **Healthy Fat Sources**: Healthy fat sources include avocados, nuts, seeds, olive oil, and fatty fish like salmon. These foods contain monounsaturated and polyunsaturated fats, which are beneficial for heart health. Limit the intake of saturated and trans fats found in processed foods, fried items, and high-fat meats.

2. **Portion Control**: While healthy fats are important, they are also high in calories. It is crucial to consume them in appropriate portions. Aim for a thumb-sized serving of healthy fats in each meal, such as adding sliced avocado to a salad or drizzling olive oil over cooked vegetables.

Meal Planning Tips

To balance macronutrients effectively, consider the following meal planning tips:

1. **Include a variety of foods**: Incorporate a diverse range of fruits, vegetables, whole grains, lean proteins, and healthy fats into meals. This ensures a wide spectrum of nutrients and flavors.

2. **Mindful portion sizes**: Pay attention to portion sizes to avoid overeating and ensure a balanced intake of macronutrients. Using measuring cups, food scales, or visual cues can help gauge appropriate portions.

3. **Plan ahead**: Planning meals in advance helps ensure a balanced distribution of macronutrients throughout the day. Consider prepping meals and snacks to have on hand, making it easier to follow a balanced diet and avoid relying on unhealthy convenience foods.

4. **Experiment with recipes**: Get creative with meal preparation by trying new recipes that incorporate a variety of macronutrients. Look for dishes that combine whole grains, vegetables, lean proteins, and healthy fats to create balanced and flavorful meals.

5. **Listen to your body**: Pay attention to how your

body responds to different macronutrient ratios. Everyone's nutritional needs are unique, so it's essential to listen to your body's signals of hunger, fullness, and energy levels. Adjust your macronutrient balance accordingly to support your individual needs and goals.

6. **Seek professional guidance**: If you have specific dietary requirements, health concerns, or goals, consulting a registered dietitian or nutritionist can provide personalized guidance on balancing macronutrients in each meal. They can help create a meal plan that caters to your needs and ensures optimal nutrient intake.

Remember, balancing macronutrients is not about strict rules or deprivation but about nourishing your body with a well-rounded diet. By including a variety of carbohydrates, proteins, and fats in each meal, you can enjoy a satisfying and nutritionally balanced eating pattern that supports your overall health and wellness goals.

CHAPTER 2: PSMF DIET RECIPES

High-Protein Omelet with Vegetables

Description: Start your day with a nutritious and protein-packed omelet filled with colorful vegetables. This omelet is a perfect combination of flavors and textures that will keep you satisfied and energized throughout the morning.

Ingredients:

- 3 large eggs
- 1/4 cup diced bell peppers (any color)
- 1/4 cup diced onions
- 1/4 cup sliced mushrooms
- 1/4 cup chopped spinach
- 2 tablespoons shredded cheddar cheese
- Salt and pepper to taste
- Cooking spray or olive oil for the pan

Instructions:

1. In a mixing bowl, beat the eggs until well combined. Season with salt and pepper.

2. Heat a non-stick skillet over medium heat and coat it with cooking spray or a small amount of

olive oil.

3. Add the diced bell peppers, onions, and mushrooms to the skillet. Sauté for 2-3 minutes until they begin to soften.

4. Add the chopped spinach to the skillet and cook for an additional minute until wilted.

5. Pour the beaten eggs into the skillet, making sure they cover the vegetables evenly.

6. Cook the omelet for 2-3 minutes or until the edges start to set.

7. Sprinkle the shredded cheddar cheese evenly over the omelet.

8. Carefully fold the omelet in half using a spatula and cook for another minute until the cheese is melted and the eggs are fully cooked.

9. Slide the omelet onto a plate and serve hot.

Nutritional Information: This high-protein omelet is a great source of essential nutrients. It provides approximately 300 calories, 20 grams of protein, 10 grams of carbohydrates, and 20 grams of healthy fats.

Greek Yogurt with Berries and Almonds

Description: Indulge in a refreshing and protein-rich Greek yogurt bowl topped with sweet berries and crunchy almonds. This combination not only satisfies your taste buds but also provides a nutritious start to your day.

Ingredients:

- 1 cup Greek yogurt

- 1/2 cup mixed berries (strawberries, blueberries, raspberries)

- 2 tablespoons slivered almonds
- 1 teaspoon honey (optional)

Instructions:

1. In a bowl, spoon the Greek yogurt as the base.
2. Arrange the mixed berries on top of the yogurt.
3. Sprinkle the slivered almonds over the berries.
4. Drizzle a teaspoon of honey over the yogurt and toppings if desired.
5. Stir gently to combine all the ingredients.
6. Enjoy this delightful and protein-packed Greek yogurt bowl.

Nutritional Information: This Greek yogurt bowl provides a healthy balance of macronutrients. It contains approximately 250 calories, 15 grams of protein, 20 grams of carbohydrates, and 10 grams of healthy fats.

Scrambled Eggs with Lean Turkey Bacon

Description: Start your day with a protein-packed breakfast by enjoying delicious scrambled eggs with lean turkey bacon. This satisfying meal is a perfect balance of flavors and will keep you energized throughout the morning.

Ingredients:

- 3 large eggs
- 2 slices of lean turkey bacon, chopped
- 1/4 cup diced onions
- 1/4 cup diced bell peppers (any color)
- Salt and pepper to taste

- Cooking spray or olive oil for the pan

Instructions:

1. In a bowl, whisk the eggs until well beaten. Season with salt and pepper.

2. Heat a non-stick skillet over medium heat and coat it with cooking spray or a small amount of olive oil.

3. Add the chopped turkey bacon to the skillet and cook until crispy.

4. Remove the bacon from the skillet and set it aside on a paper towel-lined plate.

5. In the same skillet, add the diced onions and bell peppers. Sauté for 2-3 minutes until they become tender.

6. Pour the beaten eggs into the skillet, stirring gently to scramble them with the vegetables.

7. Cook the eggs, stirring occasionally, until they reach your desired level of doneness.

8. Stir in the cooked turkey bacon, mixing it evenly throughout the scrambled eggs.

9. Remove the skillet from heat and transfer the scrambled eggs to a plate.

10. Serve hot and enjoy!

Nutritional Information: This protein-rich scrambled eggs with lean turkey bacon provides approximately 250 calories, 20 grams of protein, 5 grams of carbohydrates, and 15 grams of healthy fats.

Grilled Chicken Breast Salad with Mixed Greens

Description: Indulge in a refreshing and nutritious grilled chicken breast salad that combines the goodness of lean protein with a variety of mixed greens. This salad is a perfect option for a light and satisfying lunch or dinner.

Ingredients:

- 4 ounces grilled chicken breast, sliced
- 2 cups mixed greens (spinach, lettuce, arugula)
- 1/4 cup cherry tomatoes, halved
- 1/4 cup sliced cucumbers
- 2 tablespoons diced red onions
- 2 tablespoons crumbled feta cheese
- 2 tablespoons balsamic vinaigrette dressing

Instructions:

1. In a large bowl, combine the mixed greens, cherry tomatoes, sliced cucumbers, and diced red onions.
2. Drizzle the balsamic vinaigrette dressing over the salad and toss to coat the ingredients evenly.
3. Add the sliced grilled chicken breast on top of the salad.
4. Sprinkle the crumbled feta cheese over the salad as a finishing touch.
5. Serve the grilled chicken breast salad as a light and nutritious meal option.

Nutritional Information: This grilled chicken breast salad provides approximately 300 calories, 30 grams of protein, 10 grams of carbohydrates, and 15 grams of healthy fats.

Shrimp and Vegetable Stir-Fry

Description: Indulge in a delicious and healthy shrimp and vegetable stir-fry that combines the succulent flavors of shrimp with a colorful array of fresh vegetables. This stir-fry is packed with protein, vitamins, and minerals, making it a perfect choice for a wholesome dinner.

Ingredients:

- 8 ounces shrimp, peeled and deveined
- 2 tablespoons low-sodium soy sauce
- 1 tablespoon sesame oil
- 1 clove garlic, minced
- 1 teaspoon grated ginger
- 1 cup sliced bell peppers (any color)
- 1 cup sliced zucchini
- 1 cup sliced mushrooms
- 1 cup broccoli florets
- Salt and pepper to taste
- Cooked brown rice for serving (optional)

Instructions:

1. In a small bowl, whisk together the soy sauce, sesame oil, minced garlic, and grated ginger. Set aside.

2. Heat a large skillet or wok over medium-high heat.

3. Add the shrimp to the skillet and cook for 2-3 minutes until they turn pink and opaque. Remove the shrimp from the skillet and set aside.

4. In the same skillet, add the sliced bell peppers, zucchini, mushrooms, and broccoli florets. Stir-fry for 3-4 minutes until the vegetables are

tender-crisp.

5. Return the shrimp to the skillet and pour the sauce over the shrimp and vegetables. Toss everything together to coat evenly.

6. Cook for an additional 1-2 minutes until the shrimp are heated through and the sauce has thickened slightly.

7. Season with salt and pepper to taste.

8. Serve the shrimp and vegetable stir-fry as is or over cooked brown rice for a complete meal.

Nutritional Information: This shrimp and vegetable stir-fry is a nutritious option, providing approximately 250 calories, 20 grams of protein, 15 grams of carbohydrates, and 10 grams of healthy fats.

Turkey Lettuce Wraps with Avocado and Tomato

Description: Enjoy a light and satisfying meal with these flavorful turkey lettuce wraps filled with creamy avocado and juicy tomatoes. These wraps are not only delicious but also packed with lean protein and healthy fats.

Ingredients:

- 8 ounces lean ground turkey
- 1 tablespoon olive oil
- 1 clove garlic, minced
- 1/4 cup diced onions
- 1/4 teaspoon cumin
- 1/4 teaspoon chili powder
- Salt and pepper to taste

- Lettuce leaves for wrapping
- 1 ripe avocado, sliced
- 1 ripe tomato, sliced

Instructions:

1. Heat olive oil in a skillet over medium heat.
2. Add the minced garlic and diced onions to the skillet. Sauté until the onions are translucent.
3. Add the ground turkey to the skillet and cook until it is browned and cooked through.
4. Stir in the cumin, chili powder, salt, and pepper. Cook for an additional 1-2 minutes to allow the flavors to meld.
5. Remove the skillet from heat and let the turkey mixture cool slightly.
6. Arrange the lettuce leaves on a platter.
7. Spoon the turkey mixture onto each lettuce leaf.
8. Top with sliced avocado and tomato.
9. Roll the lettuce leaves tightly to form wraps.
10. Serve the turkey lettuce wraps as a light and flavorful meal.

Nutritional Information: These turkey lettuce wraps with avocado and tomato provide approximately 200 calories, 15 grams of protein, 10 grams of carbohydrates, and 10 grams of healthy fats.

Baked Salmon with Lemon and Asparagus

Description: Delight in a flavorful and nutritious meal with this baked salmon seasoned with zesty lemon and accompanied by tender asparagus. This dish is not only a feast for the senses but also a fantastic source of omega-3 fatty acids and vitamins.

Ingredients:

- 2 salmon fillets
- 1 lemon, sliced
- 1 bunch asparagus, trimmed
- 2 tablespoons olive oil
- Salt and pepper to taste
- Fresh dill for garnish (optional)

Instructions:

1. Preheat the oven to 375°F (190°C).
2. Line a baking sheet with parchment paper or lightly grease it.
3. Place the salmon fillets on the baking sheet, skin-side down.
4. Drizzle the salmon with olive oil and season with salt and pepper.
5. Arrange the lemon slices over the salmon fillets.
6. Toss the trimmed asparagus in olive oil, salt, and pepper.
7. Place the asparagus around the salmon on the baking sheet.
8. Bake in the preheated oven for 12-15 minutes or until the salmon is cooked to your desired level of doneness.
9. Remove from the oven and let it rest for a few minutes.

10. Garnish with fresh dill, if desired.

11. Serve the baked salmon with lemon and asparagus as a wholesome and delicious meal.

Nutritional Information: This baked salmon with lemon and asparagus provides approximately 350 calories, 30 grams of protein, 10 grams of carbohydrates, and 20 grams of healthy fats.

Lean Beef Stir-Fry with Broccoli and Bell Peppers

Description: Enjoy a satisfying and flavorful lean beef stir-fry loaded with nutritious broccoli and colorful bell peppers. This dish is a fantastic way to incorporate lean protein and vegetables into your meal while tantalizing your taste buds.

Ingredients:

- 8 ounces lean beef, thinly sliced
- 2 tablespoons low-sodium soy sauce
- 1 tablespoon oyster sauce
- 1 teaspoon cornstarch
- 1 tablespoon vegetable oil
- 2 cloves garlic, minced
- 1 teaspoon grated ginger
- 2 cups broccoli florets
- 1 cup sliced bell peppers (any color)
- Salt and pepper to taste
- Cooked brown rice for serving (optional)

Instructions:

1. In a bowl, whisk together the soy sauce, oyster sauce, and cornstarch. Set aside.

2. Heat the vegetable oil in a large skillet or wok over medium-high heat.

3. Add the minced garlic and grated ginger to the skillet. Sauté for 1 minute until fragrant.

4. Add the thinly sliced beef to the skillet and stir-fry until it is browned and cooked to your desired level of doneness.

5. Remove the beef from the skillet and set it aside.

6. In the same skillet, add the broccoli florets and sliced bell peppers. Stir-fry for 3-4 minutes until the vegetables are tender-crisp.

7. Return the beef to the skillet and pour the sauce mixture over the beef and vegetables. Toss everything together to coat evenly.

8. Cook for an additional 1-2 minutes until the sauce has thickened slightly.

9. Season with salt and pepper to taste.

10. Serve the lean beef stir-fry with broccoli and bell peppers as is or over cooked brown rice for a complete meal.

Nutritional Information: This lean beef stir-fry with broccoli and bell peppers provides approximately 300 calories, 25 grams of protein, 15 grams of carbohydrates, and 15 grams

Grilled Chicken Skewers with Zucchini and Mushrooms

Description: Indulge in the flavors of tender grilled chicken skewers paired with juicy zucchini and savory mushrooms.

This dish is not only delicious but also a great source of lean protein and essential nutrients.

Ingredients:

- 2 boneless, skinless chicken breasts, cut into chunks
- 1 zucchini, sliced into rounds
- 8-10 button mushrooms
- 2 tablespoons olive oil
- 2 cloves garlic, minced
- 1 teaspoon dried herbs (such as rosemary or thyme)
- Salt and pepper to taste
- Wooden or metal skewers

Instructions:

1. Preheat the grill to medium-high heat.
2. If using wooden skewers, soak them in water for about 30 minutes to prevent burning.
3. In a bowl, combine the olive oil, minced garlic, dried herbs, salt, and pepper.
4. Add the chicken chunks to the bowl and toss them in the marinade until well coated. Let it marinate for 15-20 minutes.
5. Thread the marinated chicken, zucchini rounds, and mushrooms onto the skewers, alternating the ingredients.
6. Place the skewers on the preheated grill and cook for about 8-10 minutes, turning occasionally,

until the chicken is cooked through and the vegetables are tender.

7. Remove the skewers from the grill and let them rest for a few minutes.

8. Serve the grilled chicken skewers with zucchini and mushrooms as a delicious and healthy meal option.

Nutritional Information: These grilled chicken skewers with zucchini and mushrooms provide approximately 250 calories, 25 grams of protein, 10 grams of carbohydrates, and 12 grams of healthy fats.

Spicy Shrimp and Vegetable Curry

Description: Delight in a spicy and aromatic shrimp and vegetable curry that combines succulent shrimp with a medley of vibrant vegetables. This curry is a flavor-packed dish that will satisfy your cravings for something warm and comforting.

Ingredients:

- 8 ounces shrimp, peeled and deveined
- 1 tablespoon vegetable oil
- 1 onion, finely chopped
- 2 cloves garlic, minced
- 1 tablespoon grated ginger
- 1 tablespoon curry powder
- 1 teaspoon turmeric
- 1 teaspoon cumin
- 1 teaspoon paprika

- 1 cup diced bell peppers (any color)
- 1 cup diced carrots
- 1 cup diced zucchini
- 1 can (14 ounces) coconut milk
- Salt and pepper to taste
- Fresh cilantro for garnish (optional)
- Cooked rice or naan bread for serving

Instructions:

1. Heat the vegetable oil in a large skillet or pot over medium heat.
2. Add the chopped onion to the skillet and sauté until it becomes translucent.
3. Add the minced garlic and grated ginger to the skillet. Sauté for an additional minute until fragrant.
4. Stir in the curry powder, turmeric, cumin, and paprika. Cook for 1-2 minutes to toast the spices.
5. Add the diced bell peppers, carrots, and zucchini to the skillet. Stir and cook for 3-4 minutes until the vegetables begin to soften.
6. Add the shrimp to the skillet and cook until they turn pink and opaque.
7. Pour in the coconut milk and bring the mixture to a simmer.
8. Season with salt and pepper to taste.
9. Simmer the curry for 10-15 minutes, allowing the flavors to meld together.

10. Remove from heat and let it rest for

Quinoa Stuffed Bell Peppers

Description: Enjoy a wholesome and flavorful meal with these quinoa stuffed bell peppers. Packed with nutritious ingredients and bursting with delicious flavors, these stuffed peppers are a satisfying option for a vegetarian or vegan dinner.

Ingredients:

- 4 bell peppers (any color), tops removed and seeds removed
- 1 cup cooked quinoa
- 1 can (15 ounces) black beans, rinsed and drained
- 1 cup corn kernels (fresh or frozen)
- 1/2 cup diced tomatoes
- 1/2 cup diced red onions
- 1/4 cup chopped fresh cilantro
- 1 tablespoon lime juice
- 1 teaspoon cumin
- 1 teaspoon chili powder
- Salt and pepper to taste
- Optional toppings: avocado slices, shredded cheese, salsa

Instructions:

1. Preheat the oven to 375°F (190°C).
2. Place the bell peppers upright in a baking dish.
3. In a large bowl, combine the cooked quinoa, black beans, corn kernels, diced tomatoes, diced red

onions, chopped cilantro, lime juice, cumin, chili powder, salt, and pepper. Mix well to combine.

4. Spoon the quinoa mixture into the hollowed-out bell peppers, pressing it down gently.

5. Cover the baking dish with aluminum foil and bake in the preheated oven for 30-35 minutes or until the bell peppers are tender.

6. Remove the foil and continue baking for an additional 5 minutes to allow the tops to brown slightly.

7. Remove from the oven and let the stuffed bell peppers cool for a few minutes.

8. Serve the quinoa stuffed bell peppers as is or top them with avocado slices, shredded cheese, or salsa for extra flavor.

Nutritional Information: These quinoa stuffed bell peppers provide approximately 300-350 calories, 10-15 grams of protein, 55-60 grams of carbohydrates, and 5-8 grams of healthy fats.

Greek Salad with Lemon Herb Dressing

Description: Refresh your taste buds with a vibrant and healthy Greek salad dressed in a zesty lemon herb dressing. This salad combines crisp vegetables, briny olives, and creamy feta cheese for a delightful Mediterranean-inspired dish.

Ingredients:

- 2 cups chopped romaine lettuce

- 1 cup cherry tomatoes, halved

- 1 cucumber, diced

- 1/2 red onion, thinly sliced
- 1/2 cup Kalamata olives, pitted and halved
- 1/2 cup crumbled feta cheese
- 2 tablespoons extra-virgin olive oil
- 1 tablespoon freshly squeezed lemon juice
- 1 teaspoon dried oregano
- Salt and pepper to taste

Instructions:

1. In a large bowl, combine the chopped romaine lettuce, cherry tomatoes, cucumber, red onion, Kalamata olives, and crumbled feta cheese.

2. In a small bowl, whisk together the extra-virgin olive oil, lemon juice, dried oregano, salt, and pepper to create the dressing.

3. Drizzle the dressing over the salad and toss gently to coat the ingredients evenly.

4. Adjust the seasoning if needed.

5. Serve the Greek salad as a refreshing and nutritious appetizer or side dish.

Nutritional Information: This Greek salad with lemon herb dressing provides approximately 200-250 calories, 6-8 grams of protein, 10-12 grams of carbohydrates, and 15-18 grams of healthy fats.

Caprese Stuffed Chicken Breast

Description: Indulge in a mouthwatering caprese stuffed chicken breast that combines juicy tomatoes, fresh basil, and creamy mozzarella. This dish is a delightful blend of flavors and textures, making it a satisfying and impressive main course.

Ingredients:

- 2 boneless, skinless chicken breasts
- 2 slices mozzarella cheese
- 2 large tomato slices
- Fresh basil leaves
- 2 tablespoons balsamic glaze
- Salt and pepper to taste
- Cooking twine or toothpicks

Instructions:

1. Preheat the oven to 375°F (190°C).
2. Butterfly the chicken breasts by slicing them horizontally, but not all the way through, and open them like a book.
3. Place a slice of mozzarella cheese, a tomato slice, and a few fresh basil leaves inside each butterflied chicken breast.
4. Fold the chicken breast over the filling and secure it with cooking twine or toothpicks to hold its shape.
5. Season the stuffed chicken breasts with salt and pepper.
6. Heat a skillet over medium-high heat and sear the chicken breasts on both sides until golden brown, about 2-3 minutes per side.
7. Transfer the seared chicken breasts to a baking dish and drizzle them with balsamic glaze.

8. Bake in the preheated oven for 20-25 minutes or until the chicken is cooked through and the cheese is melted and bubbly.

9. Remove from the oven and let the chicken rest for a few minutes.

10. Slice the stuffed chicken breasts and serve them as an elegant and flavorful main course.

Nutritional Information: This caprese stuffed chicken breast provides approximately 300-350 calories, 35-40 grams of protein, 5-8 grams of carbohydrates, and 15-18 grams of healthy fats.

Veggie-Packed Quinoa Salad

Description: Dive into a colorful and nutritious veggie-packed quinoa salad that offers a delightful combination of flavors and textures. This salad is loaded with fresh vegetables, protein-rich quinoa, and a tangy vinaigrette, making it a satisfying and wholesome meal.

Ingredients:

- 1 cup cooked quinoa
- 1 cup chopped mixed vegetables (bell peppers, cucumbers, cherry tomatoes, carrots)
- 1/2 cup cooked chickpeas
- 1/4 cup diced red onion
- 1/4 cup chopped fresh parsley
- 2 tablespoons lemon juice
- 2 tablespoons extra-virgin olive oil
- 1 tablespoon balsamic vinegar
- Salt and pepper to taste

Instructions:

1. In a large bowl, combine the cooked quinoa, mixed vegetables, cooked chickpeas, diced red onion, and chopped parsley.

2. In a small bowl, whisk together the lemon juice, extra-virgin olive oil, balsamic vinegar, salt, and pepper to create the vinaigrette.

3. Drizzle the vinaigrette over the salad and toss gently to coat the ingredients evenly.

4. Adjust the seasoning if needed.

5. Let the salad sit for a few minutes to allow the flavors to meld together.

6. Serve the veggie-packed quinoa salad as a refreshing and filling lunch or dinner option.

Nutritional Information: This veggie-packed quinoa salad provides approximately 250-300 calories, 8-10 grams of protein, 35-40 grams of carbohydrates, and 10-12 grams of healthy fats.

Grilled Salmon with Dill Sauce

Description: Treat yourself to a succulent grilled salmon fillet topped with a creamy dill sauce. This dish showcases the delicate flavors of fresh salmon and the bright herbaceousness of dill, resulting in a satisfying and healthy meal option.

Ingredients:

- 2 salmon fillets

- 2 tablespoons lemon juice

- 2 tablespoons extra-virgin olive oil

- Salt and pepper to taste

For the dill sauce:

- 1/2 cup Greek yogurt
- 1 tablespoon chopped fresh dill
- 1 tablespoon lemon juice
- 1 teaspoon Dijon mustard
- Salt and pepper to taste

Instructions:

1. Preheat the grill to medium-high heat.
2. In a small bowl, whisk together the lemon juice, extra-virgin olive oil, salt, and pepper.
3. Brush the salmon fillets with the lemon juice mixture, coating them evenly.
4. Place the salmon fillets on the preheated grill, skin side down.
5. Grill the salmon for 4-5 minutes per side or until it is cooked through and flakes easily with a fork.
6. While the salmon is grilling, prepare the dill sauce by combining the Greek yogurt, chopped fresh dill, lemon juice, Dijon mustard, salt, and pepper in a separate bowl. Mix well.
7. Remove the grilled salmon from the heat and let it rest for a few minutes.
8. Serve the grilled salmon with a dollop of dill sauce on top.
9. Pair it with your choice of roasted vegetables or a side salad for a complete meal.

Nutritional Information: This grilled salmon with dill sauce provides approximately 300-350 calories, 30-35 grams of protein, 5-8 grams of carbohydrates, and 15-18 grams of healthy fats.